AF606708

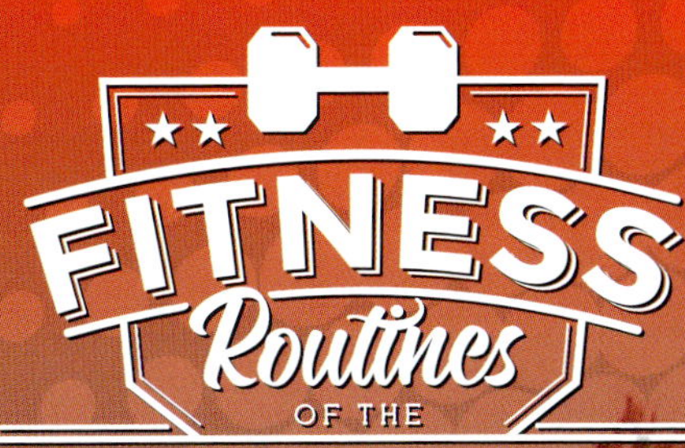

MICHAEL PHELPS

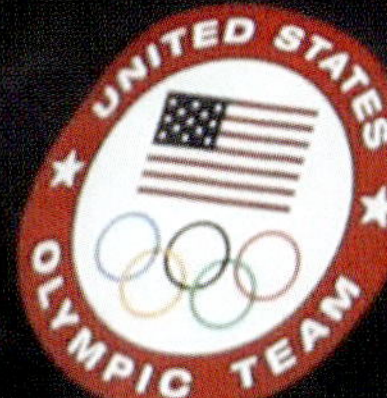

JEFF SAVAGE

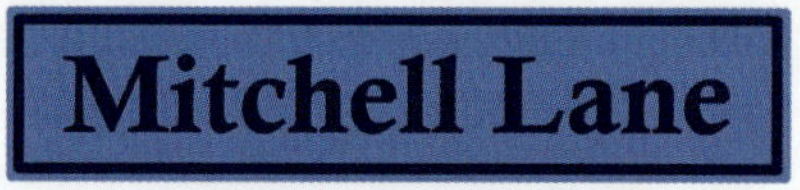

PUBLISHERS

2001 SW 31st Avenue
Hallandale, FL 33009

www.mitchelllane.com

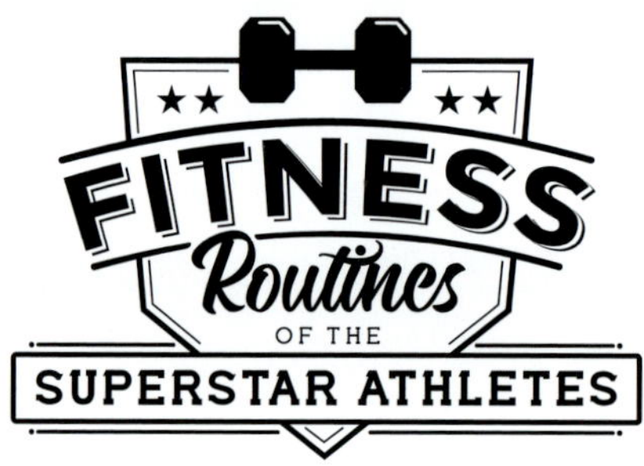

First Edition, 2020.
Author: Jeff Savage
Designer: Ed Morgan
Editor: Lisa Petrillo

Series: Fitness Routines of the Superstar Athletes
Title: Michael Phelps / by Jeff Savage

Hallandale, FL : Mitchell Lane Publishers, [2020]

Library bound ISBN: 9781680204698
eBook ISBN: 9781680204704

PHOTO CREDITS: freepik.com, newscom.com

Contents

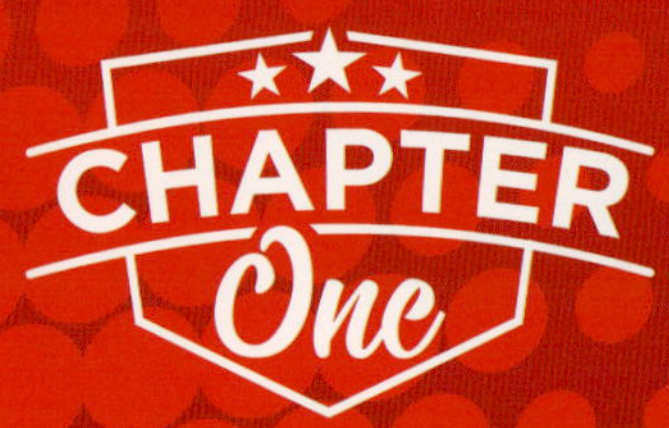

GOLD Rush

Michael Phelps blasted through the swimming pool with one billion people around the world watching. Phelps was competing in the 2016 Olympic Games in Rio de Janeiro, Brazil. He was racing seven other swimmers in the 200-meter **butterfly** event. Phelps was the greatest swimmer of all time. In other countries he was known as "Half-Man, Half-Fish." Everyone wanted to see if Phelps could make history.

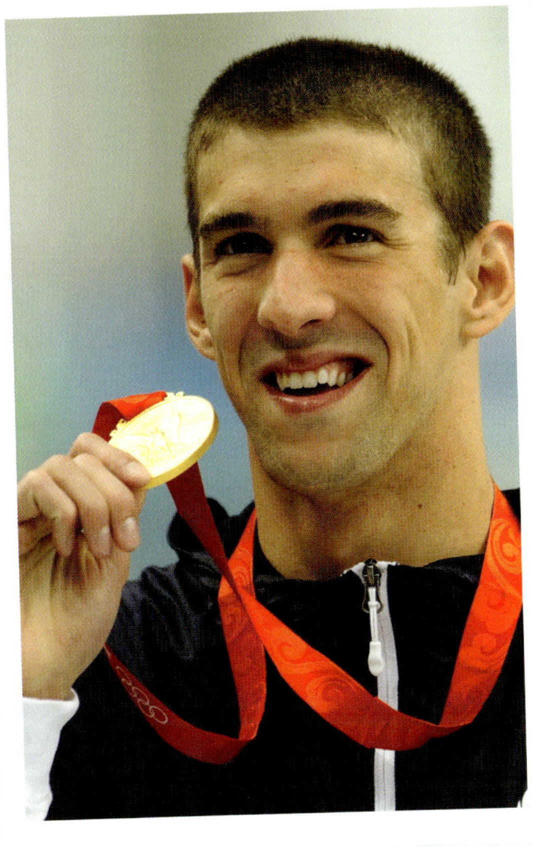

Phelps gives a smile of triumph winning his 8th medal in the 2008 Olympics.

When Phelps won his eighth gold medal at a single Olympics to break Mark Spitz's long-held record of seven first-place finishes, Spitz himself said, "He's the greatest Olympian of all time and maybe the greatest athlete who ever walked the planet." That was at the 2008 Olympics in Beijing, China—*eight years earlier*.

Phelps was now 31 years old. He was trying to become the oldest swimmer to ever win an individual Olympic gold medal. The summer Olympics are held every four years, and Phelps was competing in his *fifth* Olympics. He was 15 years old when he first raced in this event. Now he was more than twice that age. When he started his Olympic career, some of his competitors in this race were young boys who had yet to take a swimming lesson. Five of them said Phelps was their childhood hero. How was Phelps still competing?

After one lap (50 meters), Phelps was in second place behind Laszlo Cseh of Hungary. Phelps made a powerful turn and took the lead. He windmilled his arms and churned through the water with the speed of a reef shark. He watched Chad le Clos in the next lane fade away. Phelps especially wanted to beat le Clos. Four years earlier, Phelps lost gold to le Clos by a split-second. When Phelps said later he hoped to have one more chance to win the Olympic gold in this event, le Clos told him to "keep quiet." As the swimmers concentrated in the ready room for this race, le Clos jumped around punching his fists as Phelps sat in a chair glaring at him. Now Phelps was propelling past le Clos and the others. The crowd's roar at the Olympics Aquatics Center grew louder with every stroke. In just under two minutes, Phelps touched the wall first to win in a blink. Japan's Masato Sakai finished second for the silver medal. Le Clos placed fourth and failed to medal.

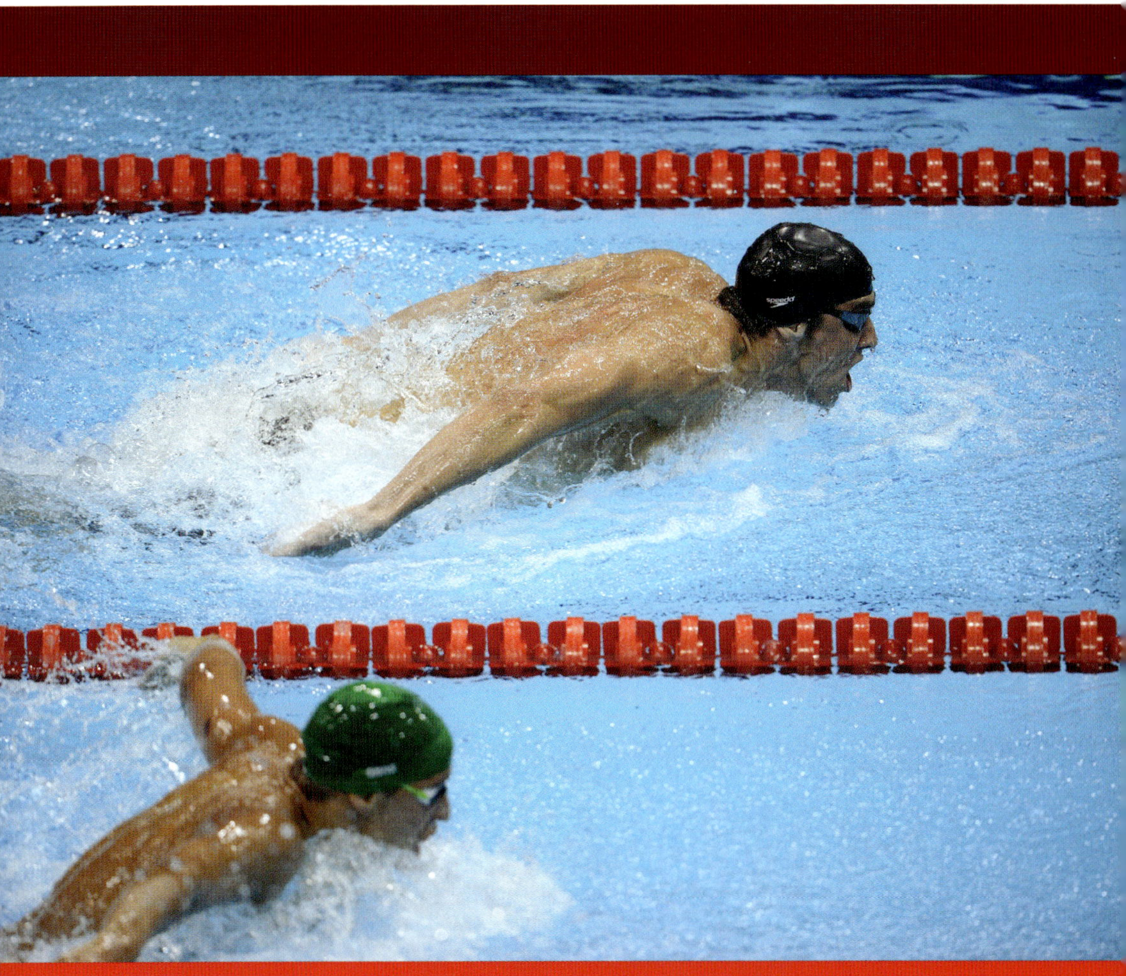

Phelps swims in the men's 200m butterfly at the 2012 Olympic Games in London, with Chad le Clos of South Africa,swimming to the left. He eventually beat Phelps for the gold.

Phelps sat on the lane rope and raised his arms in triumph. He sprang from the pool and climbed into the stands to kiss his infant son Boomer, wife Nicole, and mother Debbie. He stood on the medal stand listening to "The Star-Spangled Banner" as tears welled in his eyes. An hour later, he won another gold. Four days later, he won his sixth and final medal in Rio. It gave him 28 medals total—twice as many as any other swimmer ever and 10 more than any other Olympian in any sport. "That's a lot of medals," he told reporters. "It's insane. It's just mind-blowing to think about. I came here on a mission and that mission was accomplished. It's just really special."

Fun Fact

In 2004, a street in Phelps's hometown of Baltimore was renamed Michael Phelps Way.

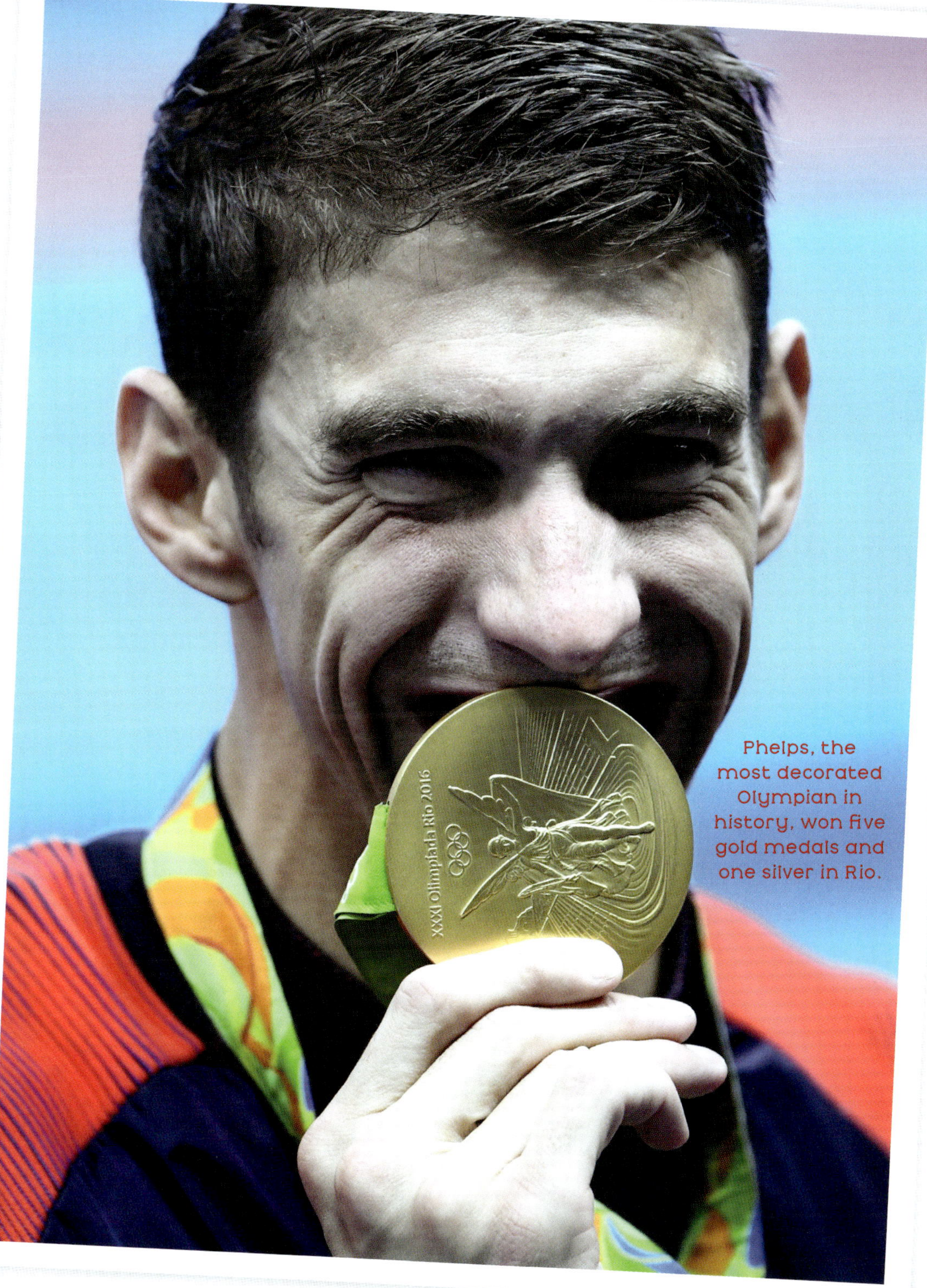

Phelps, the most decorated Olympian in history, won five gold medals and one silver in Rio.

CHAPTER Two

Breaking RECORDS

Michael Fred Phelps II was born June 30, 1985, in Baltimore, Maryland. He grew up in nearby Towson with his older sisters, Whitney and Hilary. His father, Fred, worked as a state trooper, and his mother, Debbie, was a middle school vice principal. Michael was five when he began swimming. He was afraid to put his head under water, and his instructors allowed him to float on his back. The first stroke he learned was the **backstroke**. Michael was 9 when his parents divorced and his father left home. Michael struggled to cope with his father's absence. A year later, Michael was diagnosed with Attention Deficit Hyperactive Disorder (ADHD). "He's very intense," his mother revealed later. "But he never used to be able to focus." Swimming was Michael's outlet.

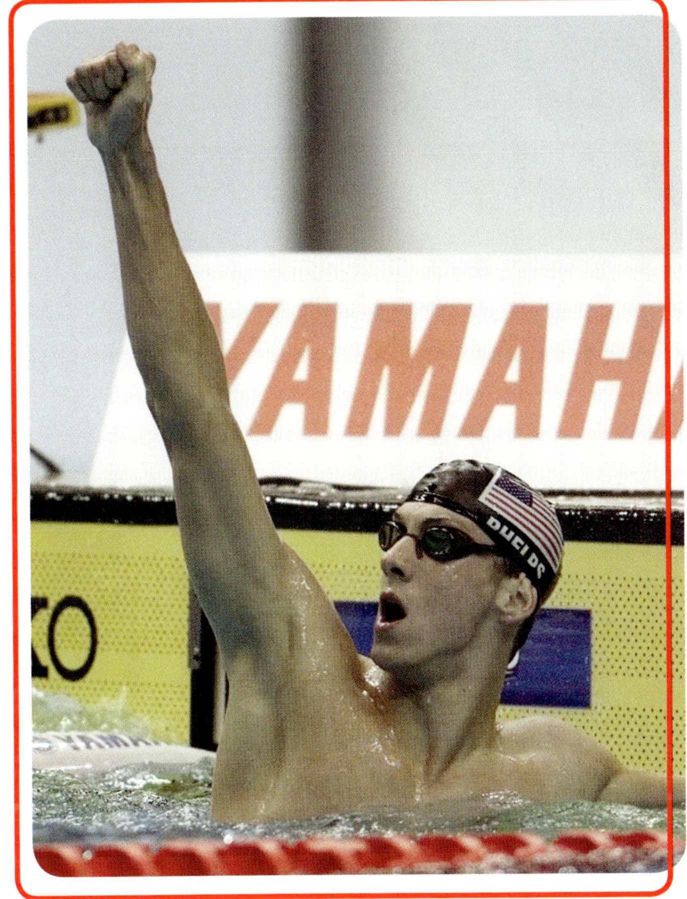

Michael punches the air after setting a new world record in the final of the men's 200m butterfly at the 9th World Swimming Championships in July 2001. Phelps set a new record time of one minute, 54.58 seconds.

Michael trained at the North Baltimore Aquatic Club and set a national record for 10-year-olds in the 100-meter butterfly (also known as "fly). In 2000, Michael became the youngest male swimmer to make the U.S. Olympic team in 68 years. He placed fifth in the 200 fly at the Games in Sydney, Australia. Early the next year he set the world record in the event, becoming the youngest male to ever set a world swimming record.

At the 2004 Olympic Games in Athens, Greece, Phelps won his first gold medal in the 400-meter **individual medley** in world-record time. He went on to capture six gold and two bronze medals—most ever by a teenager. Phelps was just getting started. Four years later, he won eight golds—seven of them in world record time. At the 2012 Games in London, England, he won six more medals to become the most decorated athlete in any sport in the history of the Olympics. By now he was one of the most famous athletes in the world. He capped his Olympic supremacy in Rio when he became the oldest swimmer ever to win gold, breaking a 96-year-old record set by Hawaiian surfer Duke Kahanamoku in 1920. How has Phelps been great for so long?

Fun Fact

Instead of wearing one swim cap, Phelps wears two. He says the extra cap makes his head feel smoother.

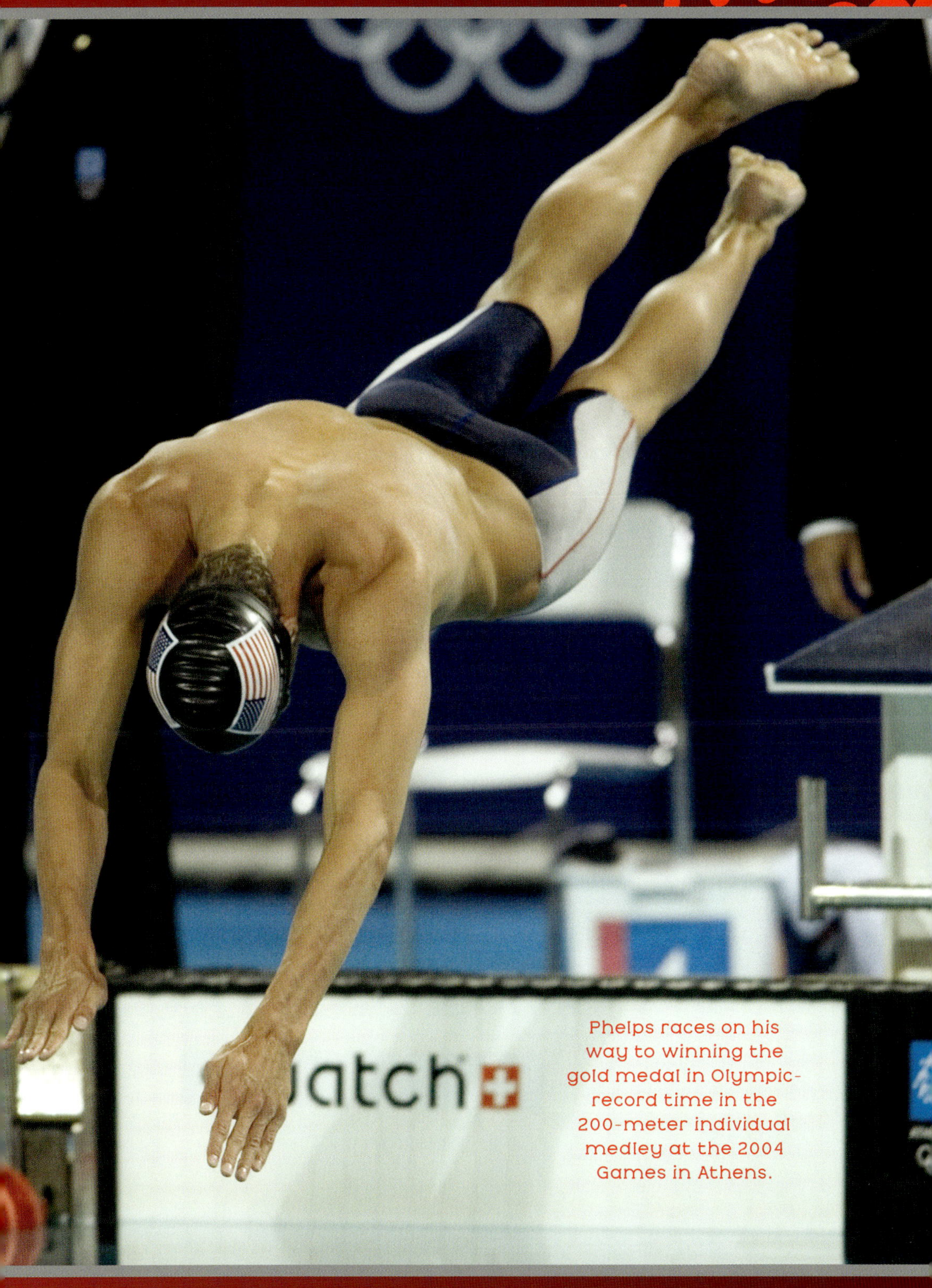

Phelps races on his way to winning the gold medal in Olympic-record time in the 200-meter individual medley at the 2004 Games in Athens.

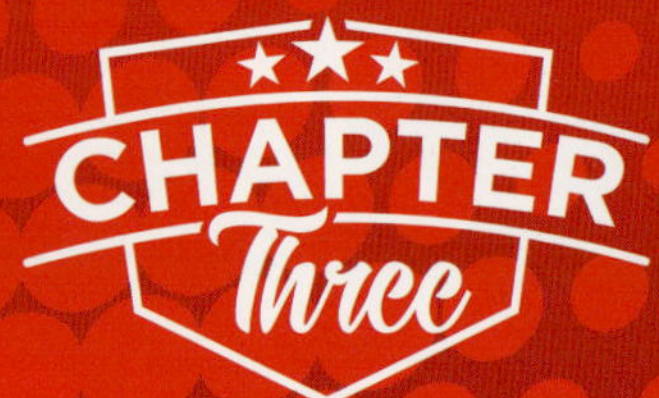

TRAINING *Machine*

No sport demands more training than swimming. Michael Phelps thrusts through the water using every muscle. His body moves with power and grace like the flow of poetry. His arms sweep as oars, his legs pound like paddles, his feet flap like flippers. His training is rigorous.

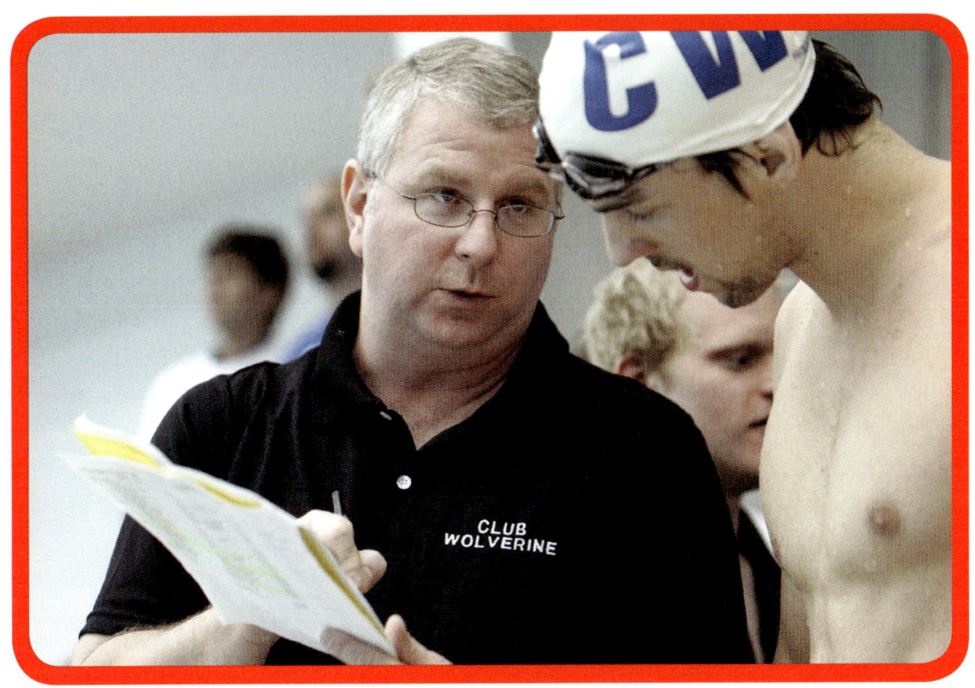

Phelps listens to long-time trainer Bob Bowman in May 2006.

Phelps was 11 years old and swimming at the aquatics center in Maryland when Bob Bowman became his trainer. Phelps said Bowman was strict like a military drill sergeant. Bowman stood at the side of the pool and barked commands—and young Phelps listened and obeyed. Several years later Phelps said, "Training with Bob is the smartest thing I've ever done. I'm not going to swim for anyone else." Phelps has been true to his word. He was still a teen when Bowman became head swim coach at the University of Michigan. Phelps moved to Michigan and enrolled at school there. Four years later, Bowman returned to Baltimore and Phelps followed. In 2015, Bowman was hired as head swim coach at Arizona State University. Phelps followed him to Arizona and lives there today.

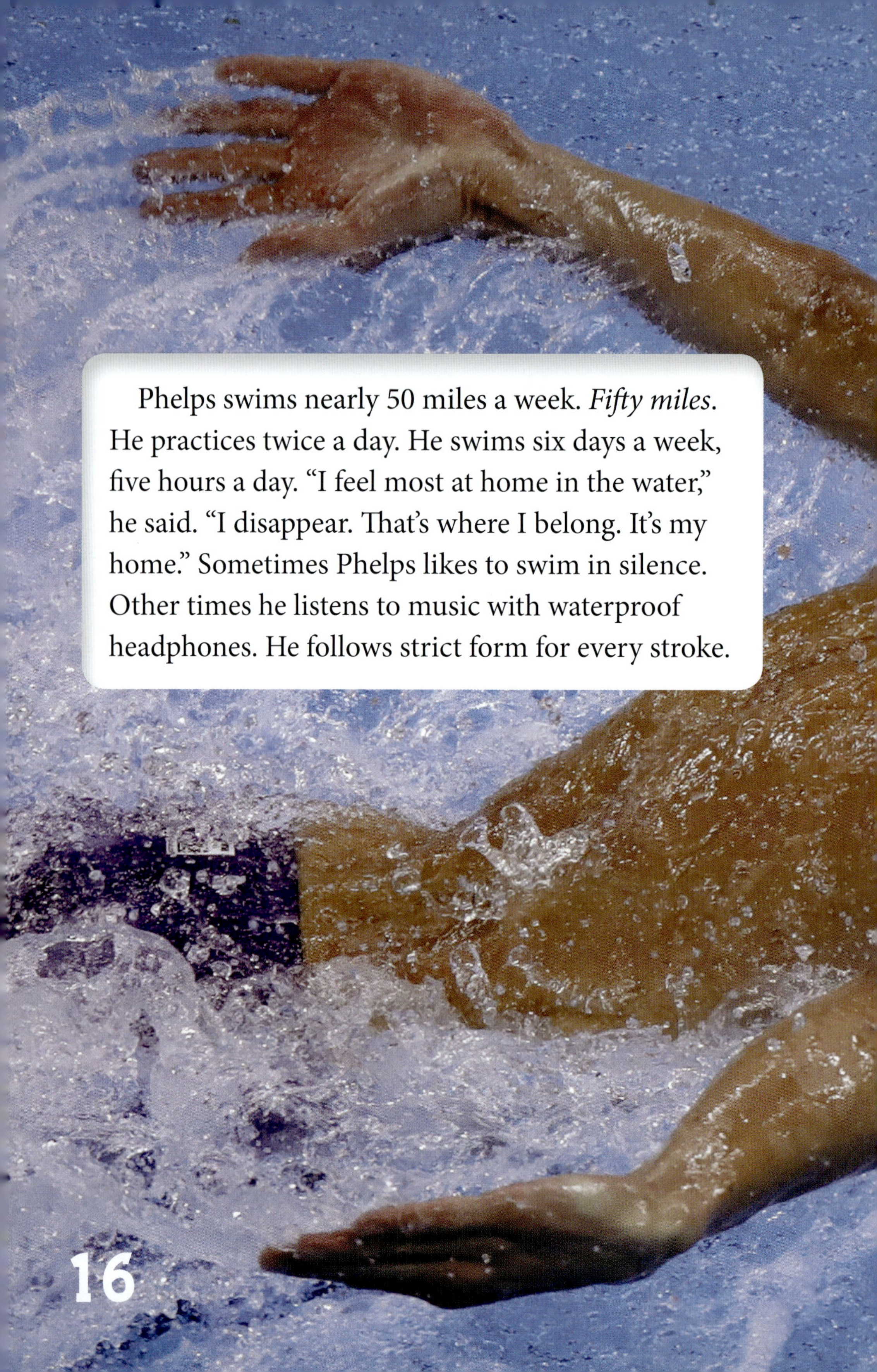

Phelps swims nearly 50 miles a week. *Fifty miles*. He practices twice a day. He swims six days a week, five hours a day. “I feel most at home in the water,” he said. “I disappear. That’s where I belong. It’s my home.” Sometimes Phelps likes to swim in silence. Other times he listens to music with waterproof headphones. He follows strict form for every stroke.

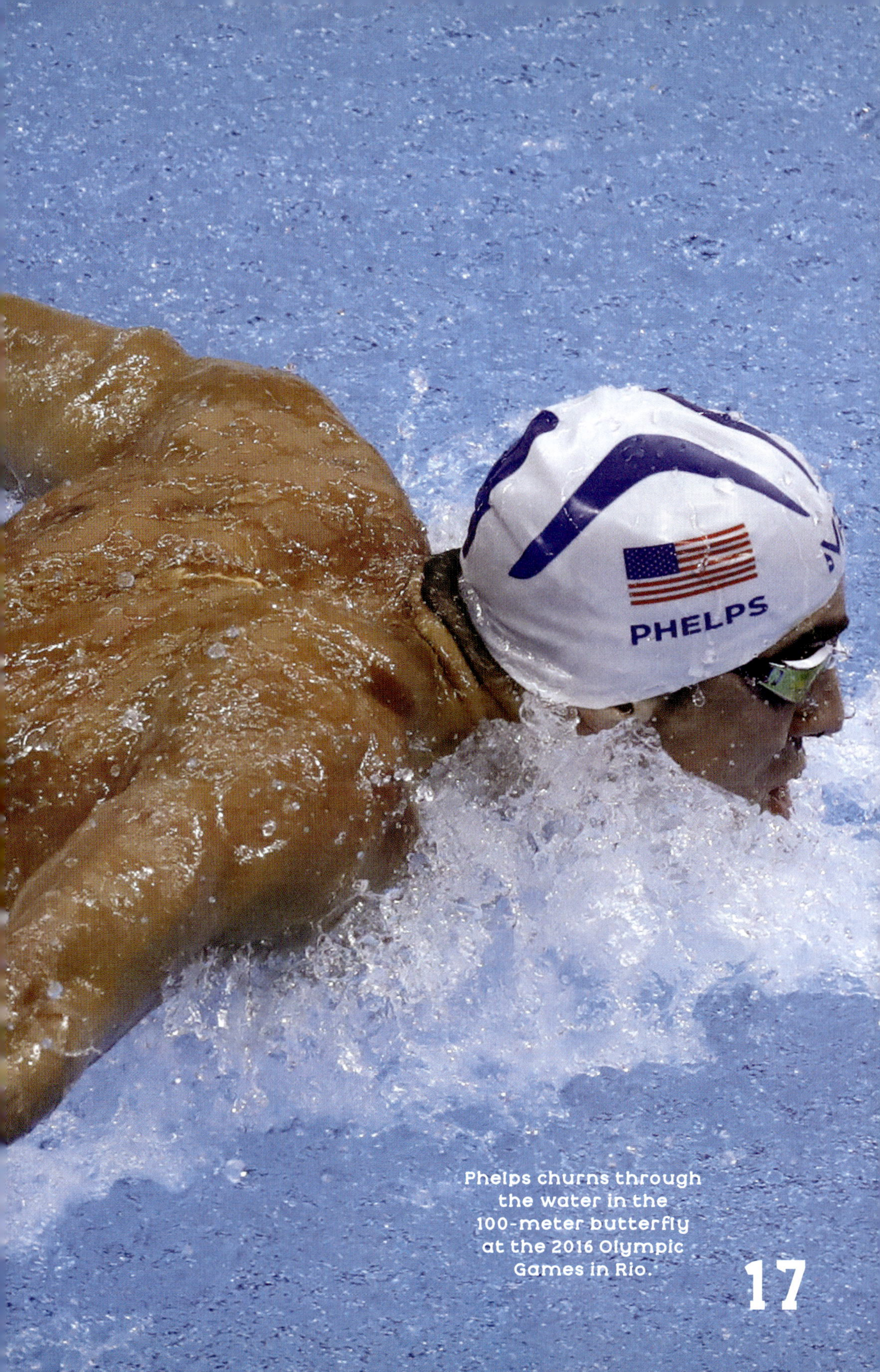

Phelps churns through the water in the 100-meter butterfly at the 2016 Olympic Games in Rio.

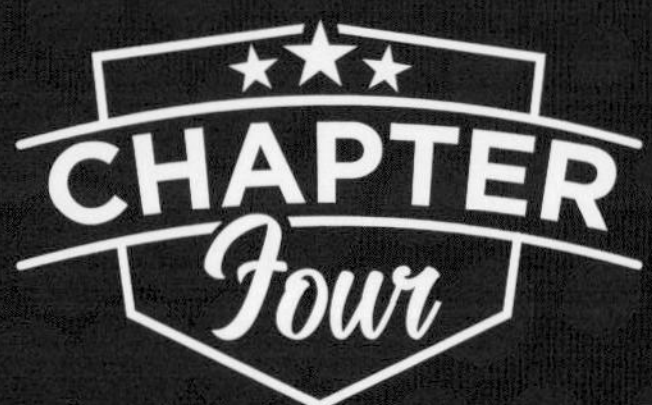

NUTRITION *King*

Phelps needs energy to train. Food provides energy. The common measurement for energy consumed and burned is the calorie. Weighing 200 pounds, Phelps would need to eat about 2,000 calories per day if he did not exercise. Phelps eats much more. In 2008, he consumed as much as 12,000 calories a day.

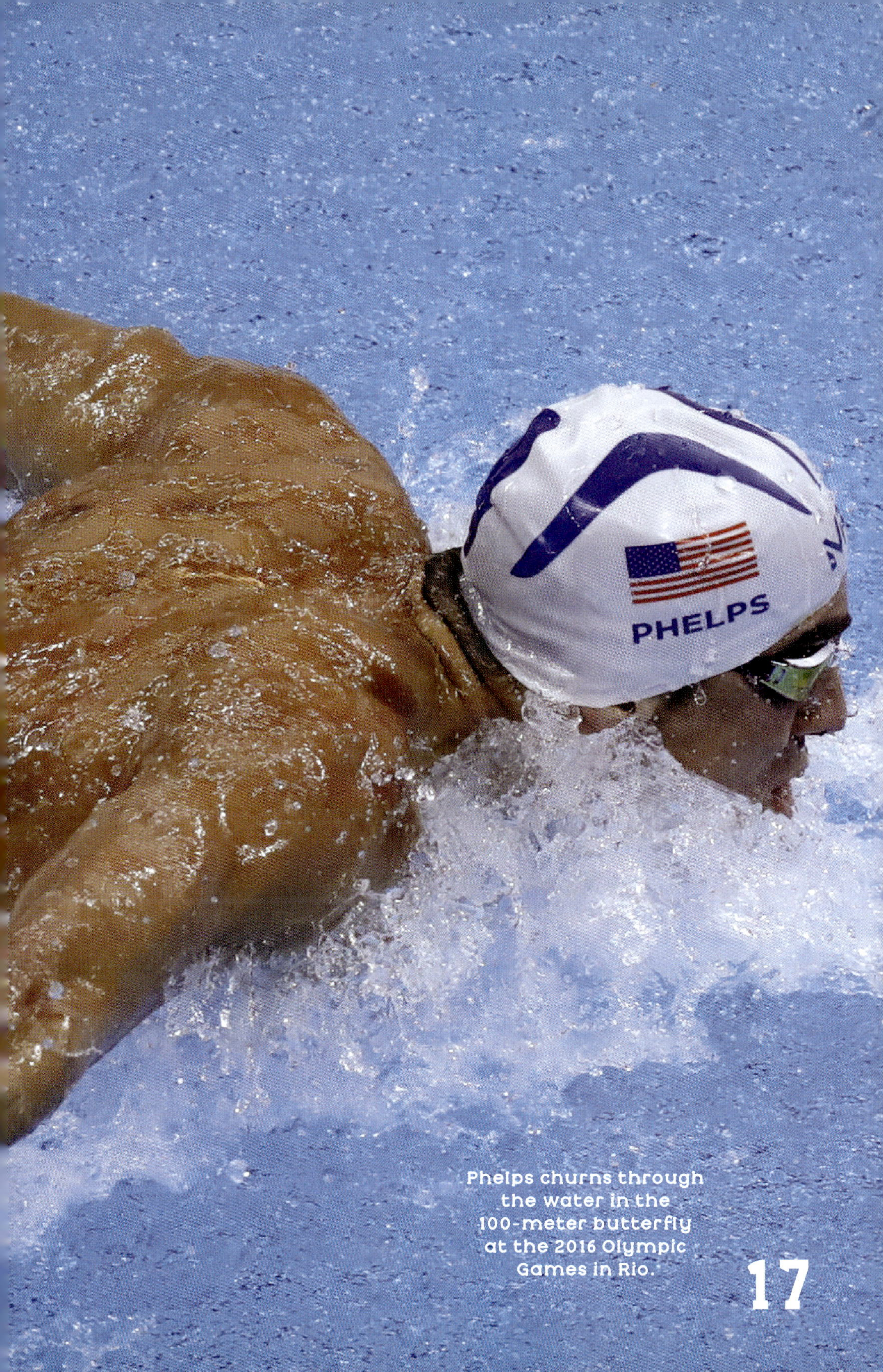

Phelps churns through the water in the 100-meter butterfly at the 2016 Olympic Games in Rio.

Phelps does multiple sets of the backstroke, **breaststroke**, butterfly, and **freestyle**. Set distances might be 50 meters, 100 meters, or 200 meters. He swims some sets at a moderate pace and others at a fast pace. Trainer Bowman pays close attention to Phelps's times. To improve his **endurance**, Phelps does long swims of 800 meters or more. To work on his **core** and lower body, he holds onto a kick board and does grueling sets of various kicks. "For me, some of the most effective drills focus on vertical kicking and underwater kicking," he told a magazine writer. "It's painful, but very effective."

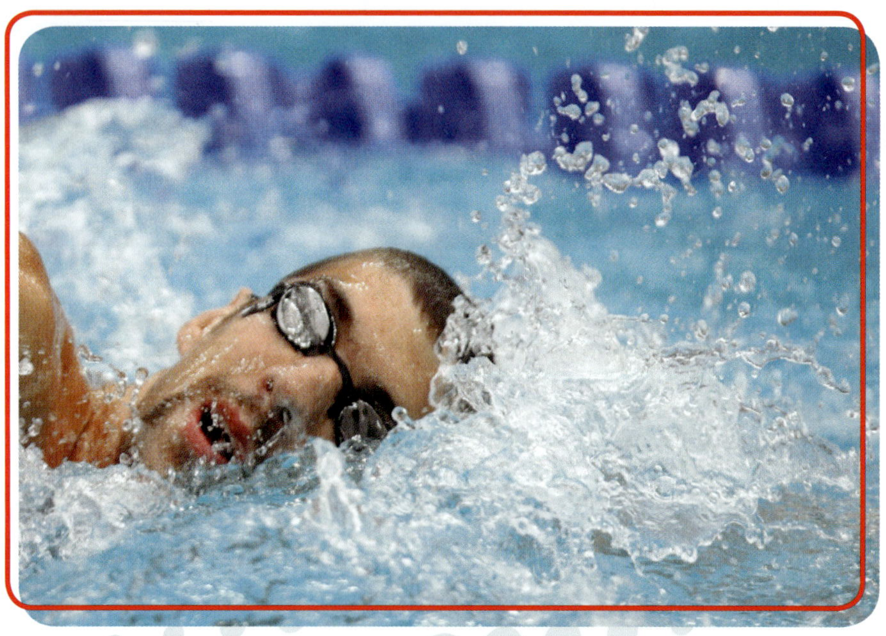

Phelps swims during a training session ahead of the Beijing 2008 Olympic Games in August 2008.

He performs a difficult stroke called **sculling** that helps him maintain his feel for the water. He does other exercises using equipment such as training paddles and a snorkel.

Swimmers call exercising out of the pool "dryland training." Phelps has increased his dryland training the last few years. He works out at a gym three days a week. He does multiple sets of pushups and pull-ups. He does three sets each of standing dumbbell **presses**, dumbbell **front raises**, and dumbbell **lateral shoulder raises**. He finishes with 500 repetitions (reps) of core exercises such as **crunches**. He also runs several miles each week.

Fun Fact

When Phelps won his 13th individual gold medal in 2016, he broke the record held by Leonidas of Rhodes from the ancient Olympics—2,168 years ago!

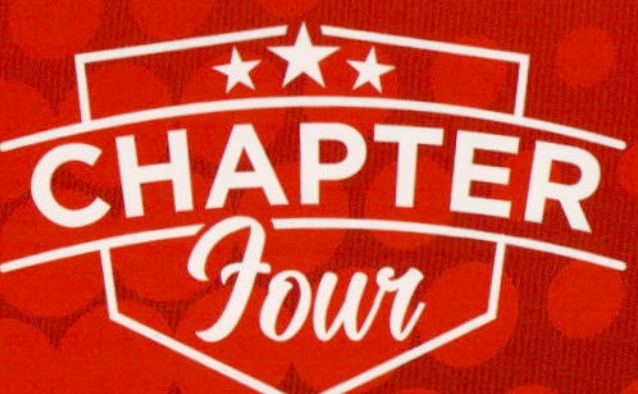

NUTRITION *King*

Phelps needs energy to train. Food provides energy. The common measurement for energy consumed and burned is the calorie. Weighing 200 pounds, Phelps would need to eat about 2,000 calories per day if he did not exercise. Phelps eats much more. In 2008, he consumed as much as 12,000 calories a day.

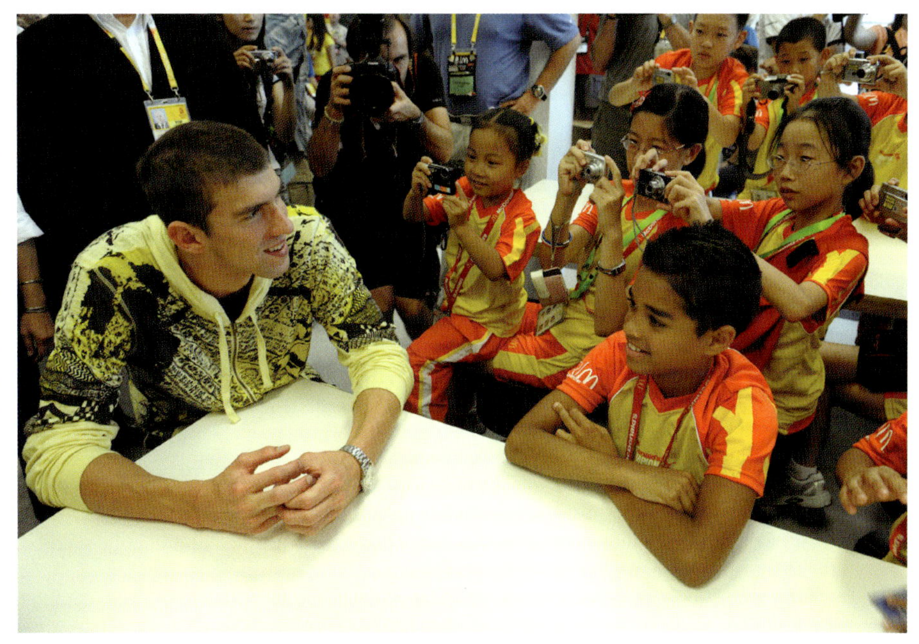

Phelps served as a global ambassador for 200 children from around the world as they experienced the 2008 Olympic Games in Beijing.

For breakfast, he ate three fried-egg sandwiches with cheese, lettuce, tomatoes, fried onions, and mayonnaise, a five-egg omelet, a bowl of grits, three slices of French toast, and three chocolate chip pancakes. For lunch he consumed a pound of pasta, two large ham and cheese sandwiches, and 1,000 calories worth of energy drinks. For dinner he ate another pound of pasta, an entire pizza, and another 1,000-calorie energy drink. "Eat, sleep, and swim. That's all I do," he told a reporter. "It's all about cramming in as many calories into my system as I possibly can. Eating is a job."

Chapter FOUR

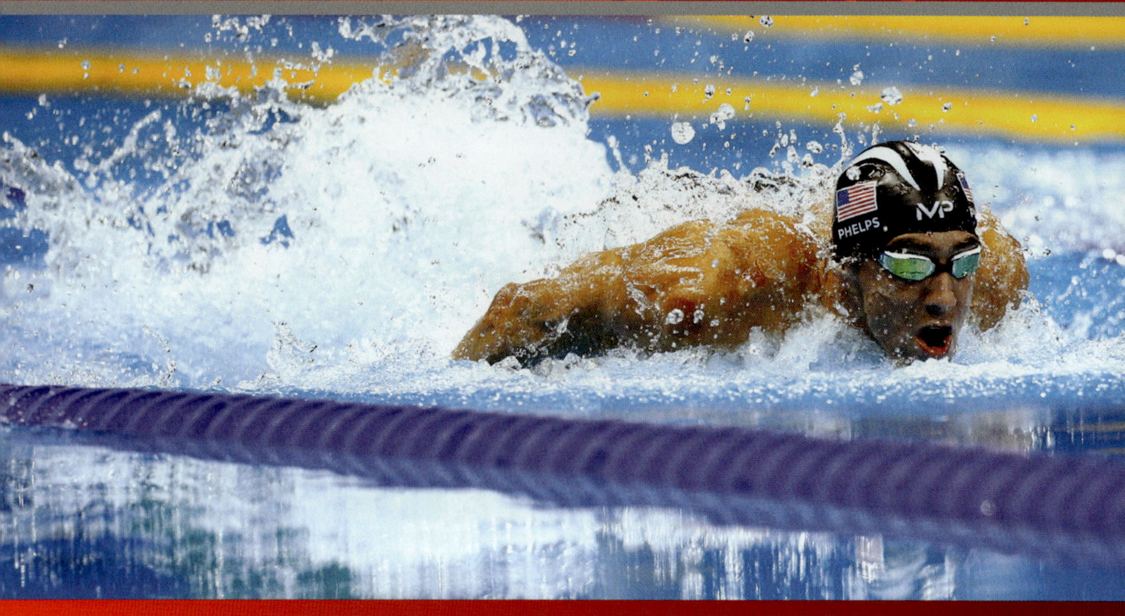

Phelps swims to the silver medal in the men's 100m butterfly swimming final at the 2016 Olympics in Rio.

By the 2016 Olympics, Phelps ate less because his **metabolism** had slowed. Still, he consumed about 8,000 calories per day. He still ate a pound of pasta for dinner, but he preferred plenty of healthy proteins, fruit, and vegetables. "I used to think that eating 'healthy' meant that it wouldn't taste good," he explained. "But now I think of my body as a high-performance car. Imagine you're a Ferrari. You're not going to put unleaded in there, you're going to put in premium gas. So if I want to get the best use out of my body, I'm not going to put bad food in there, I'm going to put in nutritious stuff that my body needs. I might have a little cheat, a cheeseburger here and there. But nine times out of ten I'm going to have chicken, fish, or a salad."

Phelps knows his body needs rest. He tries to sleep 10 hours each night. To track his recovery, he wears a device on his wrist to monitor sleep patterns, heart rate, calories burned, and other measurements. He has his blood drawn to see how his body is responding to his training.

Success at the top level of swimming requires laser focus. Phelps and trainer Bowman monitor every movement he makes in practice. This awareness gives him one more advantage. At the 2008 Olympics, when he dived from the starting block into the pool to start the 200 fly, his goggles filled with water. By the fourth and final lap, he was swimming blind. "I couldn't see, but I didn't panic," Phelps said. "I went back to all of my training. I knew how many strokes it takes me to get up and down the pool, so I started counting my strokes." Phelps won the race.

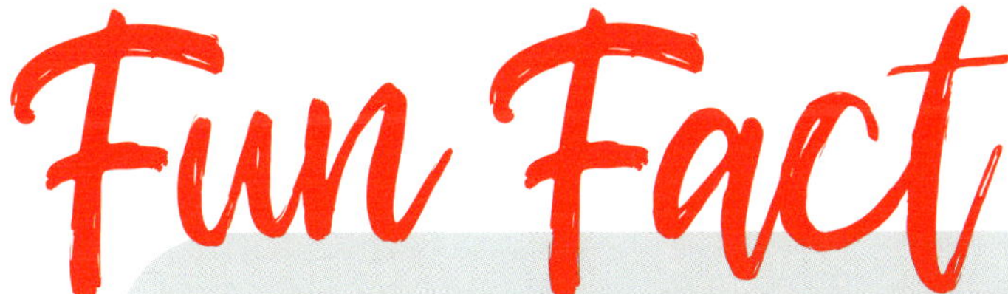

Phelps has set 39 world records—by far the most all time.

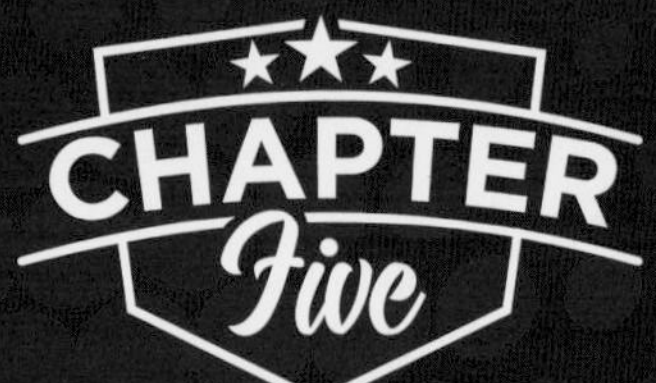

AMERICAN *Hero*

Michael Phelps is treated like an American hero. Giant parades with floats and marching bands have been held in his honor. He has been introduced on the field of pro football and baseball stadiums. His statue was placed in the International Swimming Hall of Fame *years before he was inducted.* Phelps enjoys the attention. He even agreed to star in a television program of him racing against a great white shark.

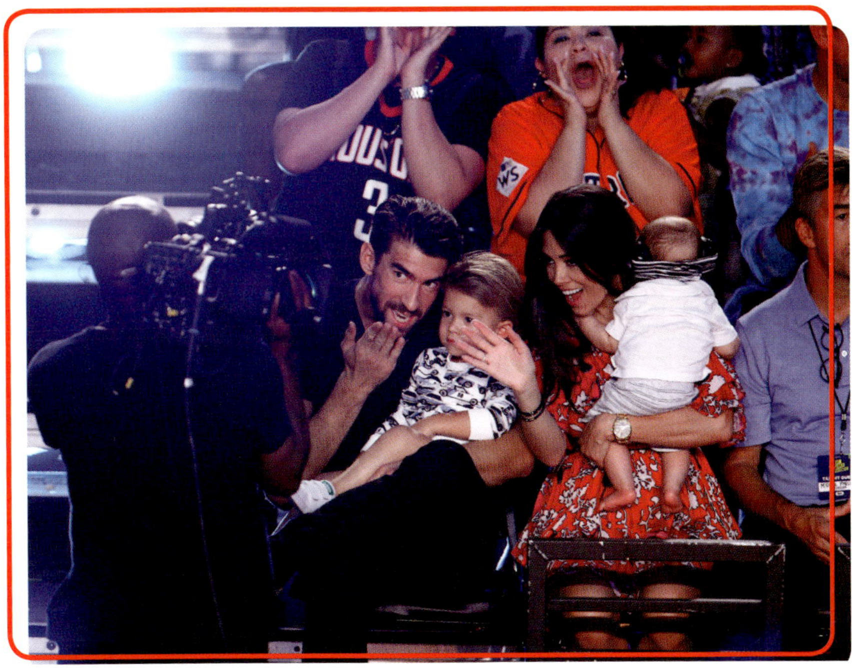

Phelps and his family—wife Nicole and sons Boomer and Beckett—attend the 2018 Nickelodeon Kids' Choice Sports Awards.

But Phelps also tries to live a "normal" life. He and his wife, Nicole, a former Miss California USA winner, are busy raising two boys—Boomer and Beckett—in Paradise Valley, Arizona. Phelps volunteers alongside Bowman as an assistant coach at Arizona State. Phelps is worth about $60 million—mostly by sponsoring companies that sell sporting goods, food products, jewelry, and pools. He gives away a lot of his money. He created Swim with the Stars, an organization that holds swim camps for children. The Michael Phelps Foundation donates millions of dollars to programs that help children learn about healthy nutrition and exercise.

Finally, there is swimming. Phelps has always found ways to motivate himself to be the best. When American teammate Ian Crocker beat him in a race in 2003, Phelps hung a poster of Crocker above his bed as a reminder. When Australian great Ian Thorpe, Phelps's hero growing up, said that Phelps could not win eight gold medals at the 2008 Olympics, Phelps taped the words to his locker in Beijing. Phelps says a positive attitude and hard work is the secret to success. "Every single day I'm living a dream come true," Phelps says. "As a kid, I wanted to do something that no one had ever done. But to be the best, you have to do things that other people aren't willing to do. Everything is possible if you put your mind to it and put the work and time into it. You can't put a limit on anything. The more you dream, the farther you get."

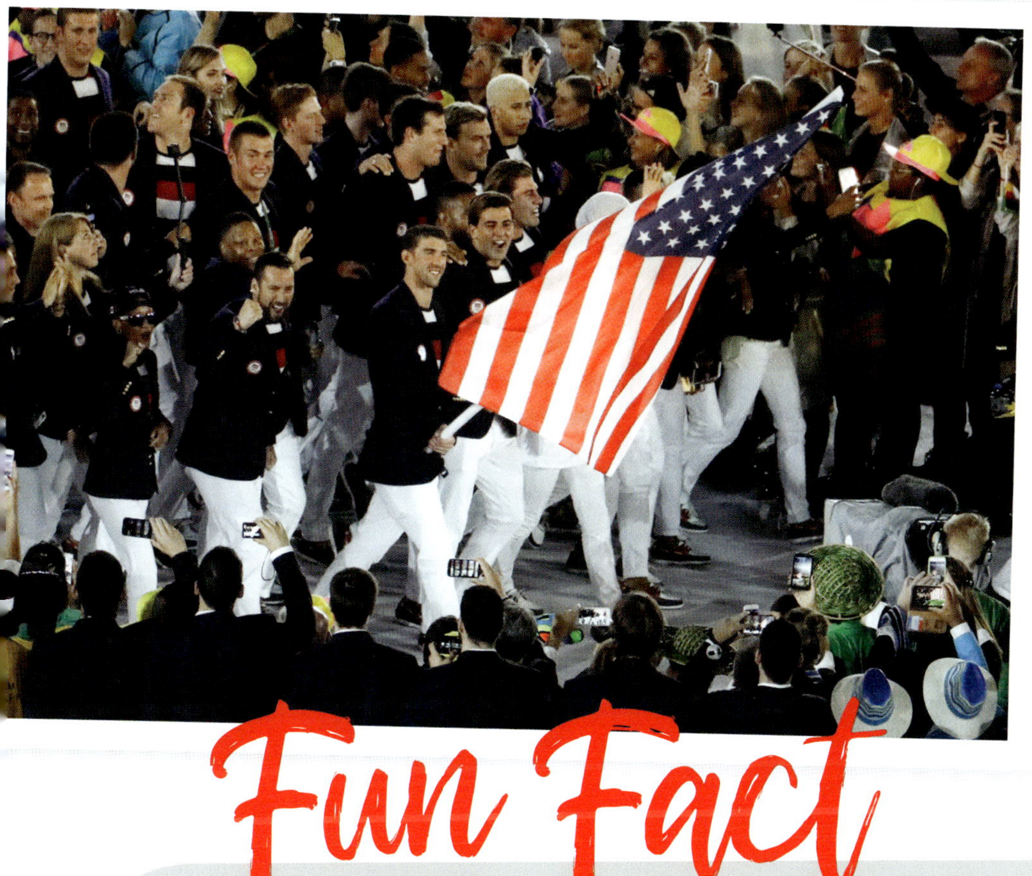

Fun Fact

At the Rio Olympics, Phelps was chosen as the Team USA flag bearer for the opening ceremony. He carried the American flag as he entered the stadium with more than 500 U.S. athletes.

AWARDS

World Swimmer of the Year (*Swimming World*)
8 times
(2003, 2004, 2006, 2007, 2008, 2009, 2012, 2016)

U.S. Olympic Committee SportsMan of the Year
5 times
(2004, 2008, 2011, 2012, 2016)

FINA Athlete of the Year
2 times
(2012, 2016)

Sportsman of the Year (*Sports Illustrated*)
(2008)

Sullivan Award (Amateur Athletic Union)
2003

Olympic Medalist
28 times

Olympic Gold Medalist
23 times

TIMELINE

1985 – born in Baltimore, Maryland

1990 – began swimming

1996 – set first national record at age 10

1996 – began training with Bob Bowman

2000 – made first U.S. Olympic team at age 15

2004 – won six gold medals at Athens Olympics

2008 – won eight gold medals at Beijing Olympics

2008 – created Michael Phelps Foundation

2012 – won four gold medals at London Olympics

2016 – married Nicole Johnson

2016 – won five gold medals at Rio Olympics

GLOSSARY

backstroke Swimming stroke performed on the back in which extended arms rotate alternately in a circular motion while legs kick in a flutter motion

breaststroke Swimming stroke in which both arms are extended forward and pull in and down while legs kick together

butterfly Swimming stroke in which both arms are extended wide and move at the same time like windmills while legs kick together

core Trunk or midsection of the body

crunches Core exercise in which you lie on your back with your knees bent and feet flat on the floor and raise your upper body slightly while holding in your stomach

endurance The ability to do something difficult for a long time

freestyle Fastest and most common swimming stroke in which arms rotate alternately in a circular motion while legs kick in a flutter motion.

front raise Exercise in which you hold a dumbbell in each hand with arms straight and raise the dumbbells forward to chin height

individual medley Competition combining the four main strokes in this order: butterfly, backstroke, breaststroke, and freestyle

lateral shoulder raises Exercise in which you hold a dumbbell in each hand with arms straight and raise the dumbbells sideways to shoulder height

metabolism The chemical process in the body that converts food into energy

press Exercise in which you hold a dumbbell in each hand at shoulder height and press the dumbbells straight up overhead

sculling Swimming stroke in which you move your arms in the shape of small figure eights

FURTHER READING

Fishman, Jon. *Michael Phelps*. Minneapolis: Lerner Publications, 2017.

Markovics, Joyce. *Michael Phelps*. New York: Bearport Publishing, 2017.

Nagelhout, Ryan. *Michael Phelps: Greatest Swimmer of All Time*. New York: Rosen Publishing, 2017.

Scheff, Matt. *Michael Phelps*. Minneapolis, MN: Abdo Publishing Company, 2017.

ON THE INTERNET

www.MichaelPhelps.com
Phelps's official site

www.teamusa.org
The U.S. national team official site

www.usaswimming.org
The USA Swimming official site

INDEX

ABOUT the AUTHOR

Jeff Savage is the award-winning author of more than 200 books for young readers. A former sportswriter for the *San Diego Union-Tribune*, Jeff's books have been read by millions. Jeff lives with his wife, Nancy, sons Taylor and Bailey, and dogs Tunes, Coach, Ace, Champ, Tank, and Lexi (that's six!) in Folsom, California. Jeff competes in triathlons, which includes a two-mile swim, but he could never keep up with Michael Phelps!